Breastfeeding
and
Bottle-feeding

an easy-to-follow guide

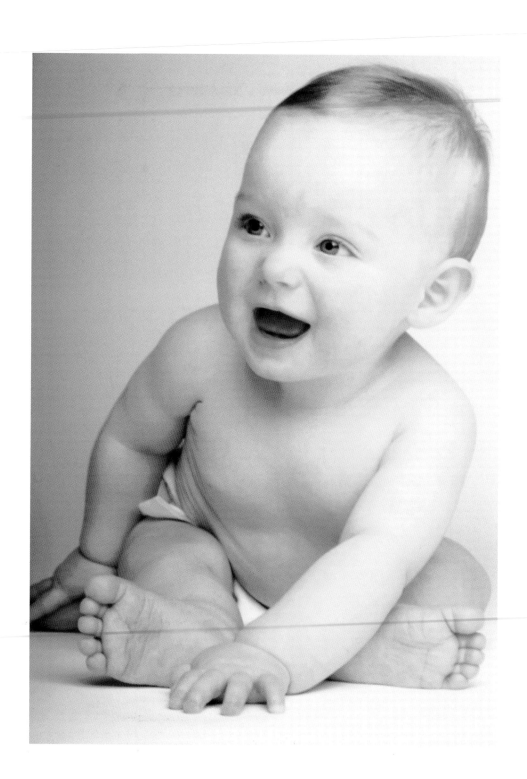

Breastfeeding and Bottle-feeding

an easy-to-follow guide

Naia Edwards

Vermilion

Contents

Introduction

Feeding your baby is one of the first things you will do after she is born and one of the most important parenting skills you will learn. It is not only essential for her survival, giving her the nutrients she needs to grow and develop, but is also the beginning of a wonderful relationship as it helps you to bond with each other. But although feeding is such a natural and fundamental part of babycare, it is not always easy. Whether you are breastfeeding or bottle-feeding, you may experience problems and find that it takes a while before you feel confident. Like most things, the more you practise the better you become at it and the easier you will find it; but there are techniques you can learn which will help to make the experience easier, and therefore more positive and more rewarding.

In this book you will find information and advice to help make feeding your baby successful and enjoyable for both of you.

Please note that to avoid confusion the baby has always been referred to as 'she' but this could just as easily have been 'he'.

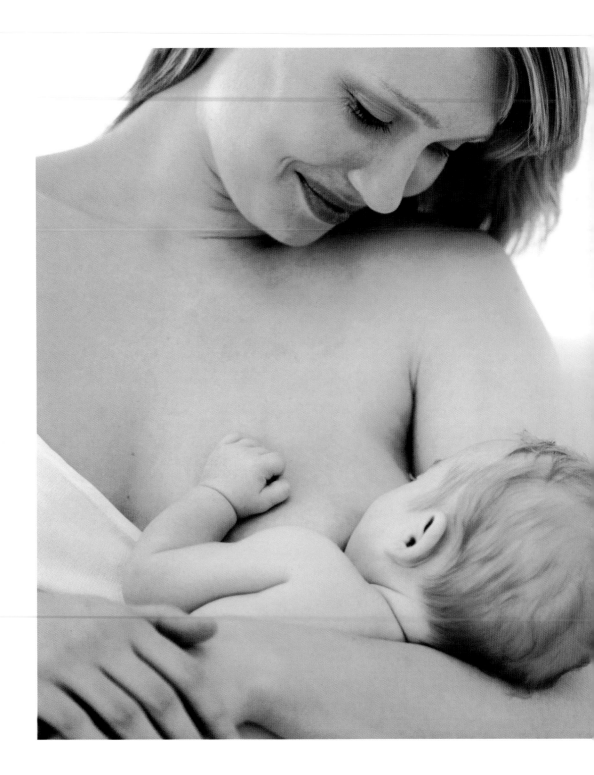

Chapter 1

BREASTFEEDING What you need to know

Whether you are expecting a baby or have just given birth, you will probably have been advised by your doctor or midwife that breastfeeding is the best way to feed your baby. At the same time you may have been told by your mother or someone of an older generation that bottle-feeding is much easier, less tiring and just as good as breastfeeding – the 'You were bottle-fed and there's nothing wrong with you' statement may be familiar to you. This conflicting advice can be confusing but exists because fashions and our knowledge and understanding of the body change over time.

Why breastfeed?

It is now known without a doubt that breastfeeding is the best and healthiest way to feed your baby. As with all aspects of parenting, however, you should always do what you feel is right for you and your baby. The official advice, from all the professional organisations – such as the World Health Organization (WHO) and UNICEF (the United Nations Children's Fund), and the UK Department of Health and Royal College of Midwives – is to breastfeed exclusively for the first six months of your baby's life. Not only is breastfeeding the most natural way, but it provides your baby with essential nutrients that formula milk can't reproduce exactly. Understanding how your body produces milk and what that milk contains may help you to make an informed decision about how to feed your baby, and see the amazing capabilities of your body!

What is breast milk?

Human breast milk is a live formula that changes according to the needs of your baby. For the first days after your baby is born, the milk you produce is called colostrum. It is full of sugar and protein for energy, and minerals and antibodies to help your baby's immune system fight off germs and diseases.

Four or five days after the birth of your baby, you will start to produce mature milk, which is made up of two parts. The first part, which your baby gets when she first starts to suck, is foremilk. This is quite thin and watery and will quench your baby's thirst. After this comes the thicker hindmilk, which is rich in nutrients and fats that are needed to help the development of your baby's brain and nervous system, and assist overall growth. The richness of this hind milk also satisfies your baby's hunger. The two parts together provide a unique food for your baby. It is tailored to her exact needs so that she will need nothing else for the first six months of her life.

How is breast milk made?

Almost from the moment of conception, your body gets ready to make breast milk – although you won't actually produce it until your baby is born. The milk is made in small sac-like glands in the breast, which are stimulated by hormones during pregnancy. From around the 20th week of pregnancy your breasts produce colostrum, which your baby feeds on for the first few days after birth; so even if your baby is born prematurely, you will be able to feed her *(see page 58)*.

Once your baby is born and starts to suck on your breasts, a hormone called oxytocin is released, which sends a release or 'let down' signal to the breast. The muscles surrounding the milk glands contract forcing milk along milk ducts to the nipple.

Within 24–48 hours of giving birth, a hormone called prolactin is released that triggers your ability to make milk. Every time your baby sucks, prolactin is released. The more the baby sucks, the more milk your body makes. This process of supply and demand means that you will always have enough milk for your baby. It also means that if you don't breastfeed and your baby isn't sucking, your body will stop producing milk.

Changes to your breasts

Whether or not you decide to breastfeed, your breasts will change during pregnancy and the first few days after your baby is born.

The first change you will probably notice quite early on in your pregnancy is that your breasts will become larger and more sensitive. For some this is a very welcome change, for others less so! The areola, the area around the nipple, also becomes larger and darker in colour. It's thought that this might be so that your baby can easily see where she needs to aim for to get fed!

Later on in your pregnancy, you may notice blue veins in your breasts; this is your body making sure that you have enough blood supply to produce milk. Small bumps around your nipples may become more apparent. These are called *montgomery glands* and they secrete an oily substance that lubricates and cleans your nipples.

Your breasts will change with the birth of your baby, and then again once you have established a feeding routine. Most women produce about 30ml (1fl oz) of milk per breast, per hour. Just before you are due to feed your baby, your breasts will feel quite hard and full; after a feed they will feel softer.

When you have finished breastfeeding, your breasts will probably go back to their original size. Some women worry that their breasts might sag. The ligaments supporting the breast tissue do become stretched while breastfeeding so sagging is possible. Wearing a good, supportive bra should reduce the possibility.

The benefits for your baby

Breastfeeding is considered the healthiest option for your baby. Here are some of the reasons why:

- Breast milk contains antibodies not present in formula milk that help your baby's immune system fight infections. These help to protect your baby from illnesses such as stomach upsets and ear infections.

- Breast milk is easy for your baby to digest and the vitamins and minerals are more easily absorbed by your baby's body. This is also why a breastfed baby is less likely than a bottle-fed baby to 'sick up' milk, technically known as possetting.

- Breast milk contains special types of fats important for the development of your baby's brain, eyes and nervous system. Adults and children make their own fats from the food they eat, but in the first six months, your baby is reliant on your breast milk to get them.

- Breast feeding reduces the likelihood of your baby suffering from allergies because it does not contain the cows' milk protein that is usually responsible for triggering them.

- Research shows that colic and excessive crying is less likely in breastfed babies. This could be because breastfed babies take in less air when they feed.

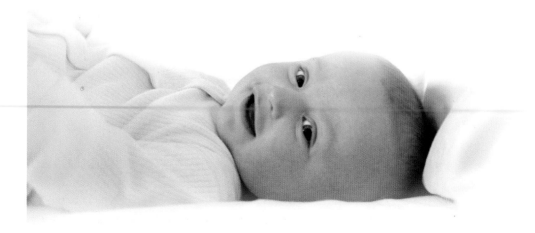

The benefits for you

Breastfeeding is also good for you. Here are some of the reasons why:

- Breastfeeding can help protect you from breast cancer and other cancers. You are also less likely to suffer from osteoporosis, a condition in which the bones become weaker.

- The hormones released when you first breastfeed help your uterus contract and shrink back to its normal size. These hormones may also help you recover from the birth more quickly, too.

- Your periods are likely to be delayed for as long as you are breastfeeding.

- The hormone oxytocin, that is released during breastfeeding, helps you feel relaxed and maternal.

- The closeness of breastfeeding may help you bond with your baby more quickly.

- Breastfeeding is the simplest way to feed – there's no need for any equipment or sterilising – and it's free!

Common concerns

Will the size of my breasts affect my ability to breastfeed?

It makes no difference whether you have large or small breasts as breast size is mostly to do with fat content rather than milk-producing glands.

Can I breastfeed if I have inverted nipples?

Again, nipples come in many shapes and sizes. Although inverted nipples or flat nipples may make it harder to breastfeed, it is still possible. Your midwife or health visitor will be able to support and advise you on how to overcome any difficulties you may experience.

Can I drink alcohol if I'm breastfeeding?

Everything you eat and drink is passed onto your baby through your breast milk so it is probably best to avoid drinking alcohol. However, alcohol clears from your milk at about the same rate as it clears from your bloodstream, so if you have one alcoholic drink just after you've breastfed your baby, it should have cleared within two or three hours, that is, before your next feed.

Does breastfeeding hurt?

Once breastfeeding is properly established the hormones released during the process actually make you feel relaxed and happy, so it shouldn't be a painful experience. However, some people experience problems with breastfeeding which can hurt *(see pages 52–54)*, but these can be overcome with the proper support.

Can I breastfeed if I've had a Caesarean?

Yes. Although you may need help picking up and holding your baby for a few days after the birth, breastfeeding will not harm your recovery from the operation. Try to use positions where your baby does not press on your tummy *(see pages 18–20)*.

Preparing to breastfeed

One of the joys of breastfeeding is that you are 'the equipment' and little else is required! However, there is a bewildering array of products on the market designed to aid breastfeeding in one way or another. Listed below are some things which you may find useful:

Feeding or nursing bras: while breastfeeding, you will find a feeding or nursing bra useful. These have special cup openings that you can undo to reveal your breast without having to undo the whole bra. There are lots of different bras available at varying prices. Try some on to find the one that is most comfortable, and then practise undoing it and doing it up again with one

GETTING A GOOD BRA

Wearing a bra that fits properly is important for the comfort and support it provides. It's worth having a bra properly fitted quite early on in your pregnancy, as soon as your breast size changes. On average a woman will gain about two cup sizes and some women may gain over 680g (1.5lb) in weight per breast.

hand. Once you have found the one you are happy with, it's a good idea to buy several.

Breast pads: leaking breasts are a natural, if sometimes slightly embarrassing, part of breastfeeding. It is very common to leak a little either during a feed or even when you're not feeding. Breast pads prevent milk leaking onto your clothes. They fit inside your nursing bra to absorb excess milk and prevent damp patches staining your clothes. Breast pads are available as either disposable or machine-washable. They are usually made of cotton and may have adhesive on one side to keep them in place.

Feeding pillow: this is a V-shaped cushion that you place around your side, with one arm of the V underneath your feeding breast and the other around your back. It helps with breastfeeding by bringing your baby up to the right height to feed and helps support the weight of your baby, which makes it easier for you to get into a comfortable position and relax. It's also good for propping your baby up before she can sit up for herself.

Breast pumps: these are machines that 'express' milk from your breast into a bottle, so that someone else can feed your baby. They are also used to increase the supply of breast milk if it is low. There are many different types of pumps available. The most effective ones are electric – they are expensive to buy, but are available for hire, too. Otherwise opt for a manual pump or try expressing by hand *(see page 37)*. Talk to your midwife, health visitor or breastfeeding supporter for more information.

Nipple shields: if you have inverted nipples, these thin plastic or rubber cups, which fit inside your bra, help push out your nipple and make breastfeeding easier. They are also used to protect sore nipples when you are feeding. Instead of attaching herself to your nipple, your baby attaches herself to the nipple shield and sucks the milk through it.

Muslin cloths: most babies will 'spit up' a bit of milk after a feed at some point. An absorbent muslin cloth worn over your shoulder, beneath your baby's chin, will help to protect your clothes.

The importance of a healthy diet

Perhaps one of the best things you can invest in for breastfeeding is yourself. It is even more important than usual that you are fit and healthy because breastfeeding uses up a lot of your energy. You need to keep your strength up. It is also important that you eat the right foods because whatever you eat will be passed onto your baby.

Tips for healthy eating: when you have a small baby, it can be difficult to find the time to eat a balanced diet and to prepare good food. Here are some simple ways to eat well:

1. You don't need to eat for two, as perhaps you may have done while you were pregnant, but it is important not to worry about trying to lose weight and dieting while you are breastfeeding. Breastfeeding burns up approximately 500 extra calories a day and you need to keep up your energy levels.

2. Try to eat a variety of foods including:

- Plenty of fruit and vegetables – aim for five portions a day to keep up your vitamin and mineral intake.

- Starchy foods – such as bread, pasta, rice and potatoes – will give you the extra energy you'll need.

- Fibre – found in wholegrain bread, breakfast cereals, pasta, and rice – will keep your bowels regular which can be a problem just after childbirth.

- Protein such as lean meat and chicken, fish, eggs and pulses, also provides energy and is important for growth and body maintenance and repair.

● Fish, at least twice a week, including some oily fish because it is high in long chain omega 3 fatty acids which are good for your joints and help reduce the risk of heart disease.

● Dairy foods – such as milk, cheese and yoghurt – contain calcium and are a useful source of protein.

3. You don't need to prepare anything elaborate. Keep meals as simple as possible and say 'yes' to anyone who offers to cook for you! Eating little and often may also help save you time as it will mean fewer large meals to prepare. Some healthy snack ideas include dried fruit and nuts, cereal bars, fruit smoothies made by whizzing up a carton of fruit yoghurt with some of your favourite fruit or fruit juice and a dollop of ice cream, and sticks of raw vegetables like carrots, peppers, celery and cucumber dipped into hummus.

4. Drink lots of fluid. Breastfeeding makes you very thirsty and you will need to drink at least 6–8 glasses of fluid a day, preferably water. Keep your caffeine intake to a minimum. It's a good idea to keep a glass of water beside you while you're feeding.

FOODS TO AVOID
While you are breastfeeding, you should avoid:
• More than one portion of shark, swordfish or marlin per week because they contain high levels of mercury which is a toxin.
• More than two portions of oily fish – such as mackerel, sardines, trout or fresh tuna – each week because they have very small levels of dioxins (environmental pollutants) which may build up in your body over time.
• Nuts and nut products – especially peanuts – if you or your baby's father, brother or sister suffers from certain allergic conditions, such as hay fever, asthma or eczema.
• If you think that some of the foods you eat are affecting your baby, talk to your GP or health visitor before cutting them out of your diet.

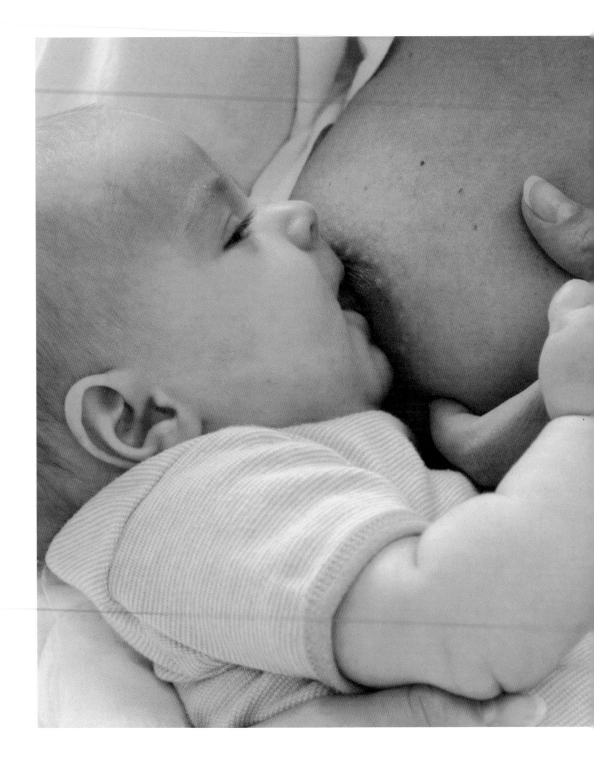

Chapter 2

BREASTFEEDING Getting started

For the nine months of your pregnancy your baby has been fed by the placenta. Now that she has arrived in the world, she is totally reliant on you. Fortunately, your breasts can produce all the food your baby will need for the next six months. Breastfeeding may be natural but not all women find it easy. It takes some women longer to establish feeding, but it is worth persevering and seeking help from your health visitor, midwife or breastfeeding supporter if necessary.

Basic steps for feeding your baby

Being prepared will increase your chances of breastfeeding your baby successfully.

Decide where you want to feed your baby: find somewhere comfortable and put your feet up, literally! You need to raise the level of your feet so that your lap is flat enough to support your baby. Use a low stool, some magazines or a cushion under your feet. Also make sure you have enough support under your arms, such as a pillow, because even a tiny baby can feel quite heavy after a while.

Get what you need to hand. You may be there for some time so it's a good idea to make sure you also have things you need within easy reach:

- Jug of water and a glass – you will find that you feel very thirsty when you start to feed and it is important to stay hydrated.

- Telephone – once you've started feeding you won't want to move to pick up a ringing phone. It won't be long before you are able to breastfeed and have one hand free for holding a phone.

- Something to read – although it is wonderful for you and your baby to look at each other while you are feeding, you can't do this all the time, especially if it's a long feed. Having a book or a magazine to look at will help the time go by.

Hold your baby in the right position: there are lots of different ways to hold your baby for feeding and you will need to find the one that feels most comfortable and natural for both of you. You might prefer to feed lying down sometimes, especially during the night, but at other times you might want to sit in a chair. Whichever position you choose, try to be as relaxed as possible and create as calming and soothing an atmosphere as you can.

Popular positions for holding your baby:

Try the following positions and use the ones you find most comfortable:

Cradle position: this is the most commonly used sitting position, for feeding a newborn baby. Using the arm closest to the breast you want to feed from, hold your baby 'tummy to tummy', so that she is turned on her side with her tummy facing towards you. Her head should lie in the crook of your arm, while your inner arm runs along her back and your hand supports her bottom. Your baby's mouth needs to be at the same height as your nipple, so it's a good idea to place a cushion or pillow underneath your arm to help support your baby. Your free hand can cup your feeding breast in a C-hold with your fingers underneath your breast and your thumb on top.

Rugby hold: so-called because you hold your baby under your arm like a rugby ball! It's actually a very good position for beginners or if you've had a Caesarean birth because the baby doesn't lie against your tummy. Firstly, put your baby on a pillow or cushion beside you with her head in front of your breast and her feet pointing behind you, tucked under your arm. Use your hand to support her head and the rest of your arm to cradle her close to you. Your spare hand is used to hold your breast in the C-hold.

Cross-cradle position: this is another popular sitting position because it gives you the most control in holding your baby. Again your baby should lie with her tummy facing towards you, but this time use the arm on the opposite side from your feeding breast to support her. Put your hand at the back of your baby's neck with your thumb and index finger behind each ear. Your free hand can support your breast in the C-hold again.

Lying down position: this is a great position for feeding during the night when you're tired or unwell, or if you have had a Caesarean birth. Both you and your baby lie on your sides facing each other, tummy to tummy. Cradle your baby in the arm closest to the side you're feeding from and bring her in close to you. Use your free hand to hold your breast in the C-hold.

YOUR BABY'S POSITION
It's important to make sure your baby is in the correct position.
• Her whole body should be facing your breast. Whichever position you are in, she should be lying on her side not on her back.
• Her back should be in a straight line, so that she doesn't have to turn her head to feed.
• She should be tucked in as close to you as possible.

As you become more confident you will find that you can feed your baby easily in any position – standing up, sitting with your legs crossed, or lying down – but give yourself some time to practise.

Latching on
Getting your baby attached to your breast is called 'latching on', and doing it correctly is probably the most important part of breastfeeding. It may take a bit of practice to get it right. Do ask your midwife or health visitor to help you and check whether you're doing it right.

Here are some basic steps to latching on which may be helpful:

● Get your baby to open her mouth as wide as possible. She needs to get both your nipple and the dark area around your nipple into her mouth. You can encourage her to open her mouth by stroking her cheek or upper lip with your nipple.

● While your baby's mouth is open, quickly bring her to your breast. She should tilt her head back slightly so that her nose is level with your nipple, but clear of your breast so that she can breathe easily.

● Aim the nipple over your baby's tongue and towards the roof of her mouth. Her tongue will press the milk out from the milk glands around the nipple.

If your baby is latched on properly:

● She should have a large mouthful of breast.

● Her chin should be touching your breast.

● There should be more of your breast below your nipple in her mouth than above it.

● It shouldn't hurt you to feed (after the first few sucks) and your milk should flow freely.

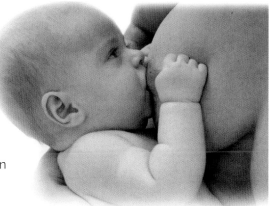

● Your baby's cheeks should be rounded during sucking.

● You should notice movement in the whole jaw as she sucks.

● Your baby should finish the feed and come off the breast on her own.

● Your baby should be calm and relaxed.

If these things are not happening and it's painful, slide your finger into your baby's mouth to break the latch and try again. Seek help from your midwife or health visitor, if necessary.

TOP TIP

A good way to get your baby to open her mouth to feed is to squeeze a bit of milk out of your nipple so she can smell it.

How your baby sucks

Your baby's sucking stimulates the 'let down' reflex *(see page 24),* which you may feel as a tingling sensation in your nipples. After the first few hungry gulps, she should settle down to a more regular rhythm of feeding. You should be able

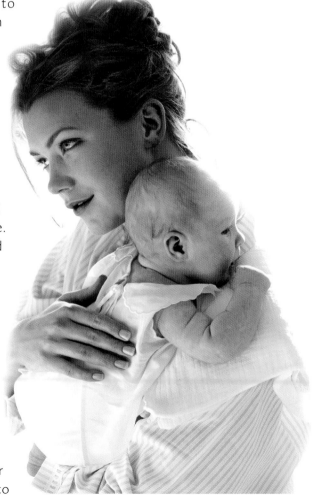

TOP TIP
Don't lean your baby over too much to burp her as this could make her sick. Rubbing or patting her too enthusiastically can also make her sick.

to hear her suck, suck, suck, swallow and then repeat the pattern. The first milk will quench her thirst. For your baby to reach the thicker energy-giving hindmilk, you must let her completely empty a breast, which may take 15–30 minutes.

If your baby is still hungry, offer the second breast. To begin with, one breast will probably be enough, but as she grows she will need more milk to satisfy her. Try to remember which breast your baby finished feeding on so you can start on the other breast next time. If you keep on feeding from the same breast, your other breast will stop producing milk.

Winding your baby

Most babies swallow a bit of air while they are feeding, which will make them feel uncomfortable. Although breastfed babies are said to need less winding than bottle-fed babies, if she is crying and you know she's not hungry, then helping her to burp and bring up the wind, might be what she needs. You might need to do this once or several times during the feed or just at the end of a feed. Your baby might not need winding after every feed, but it's worth a try because you don't want to put her down to sleep and for her then to wake up crying because she's got wind.

There are a number of different ways you can wind your baby:

- Sit her on your lap so that she is leaning forward slightly; support her with one hand spread against her chest. Rub or pat her back gently with your other hand.

- Hold her against you with her head facing over your shoulder and rub or pat her back gently.

- Lie her on her tummy across your lap and pat or rub her back.

Possetting

Most babies will 'sick up' a bit of milk after a feed; this is called possetting. Breastfed babies apparently don't posset as much as bottle-fed babies because breast milk is so easily absorbed, but it varies from baby to baby. Possetting doesn't upset your baby or cause her any harm and as your baby gets bigger and her muscles get stronger will gradually reduce and resolve itself naturally by 18 months . If your baby sicks up a lot – it can sometimes seem as though she's regurgitated her whole feed – it is usually nothing to worry about. But if you are worried, or your baby seems to be in pain, seek advice from your health visitor or GP. Keep a muslin cloth to hand to wipe your baby's face and to protect your clothes. You might also want to put a bib on your baby to protect her clothes if she is prone to possetting.

TOP TIP
To remove the smell of baby sick from cloths or clothes use a sprinkling of bicarbonate of soda.

TOP TIP
If you are having problems winding your baby, try rubbing her fontanelle very gently with your finger and this should make her burp. Strange but true!

THE LET DOWN REFLEX

The let down reflex, also known as the milk ejection reflex, is caused by the hormone oxytocin which stimulates the muscles of the breast to squeeze out milk. For the first few days after your baby is born, your baby's sucking releases the hormone. Later, anything that makes you think about your baby, or feeding your baby, can trigger this hormone release.

You may feel a slight tingling or pain in your nipple when let down occurs, or you might not feel anything at all. Everyone is different. You might become more aware of the let down when your baby is a few weeks old. As breastfeeding becomes established, you will get used to it and stop noticing it altogether.

The first time you feed your baby

No one can explain the marvel of meeting and holding your baby for the very first time. You may be feeling all sorts of emotions, and be exhausted after a long labour, but you will want to see your baby, touch her and hold her. Putting your baby to the breast soon after she's born and offering her a feed is as much a part of the process of getting to know each other as it is about actually feeding her.

If you are keen to breastfeed, you should write this down in your birth plan, so the hospital staff can help you. In most cases, your midwife will lift your baby onto you as soon as she is born and the skin-to-skin contact you have with your baby will help her to breastfeed.

Hold her close to your breast to see if she 'roots' for it – opens her mouth looking for your breast – which is a natural reflex in newborn

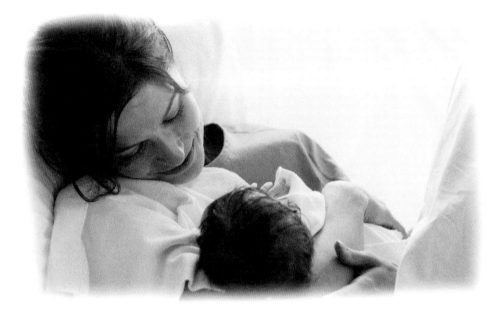

babies. If she does and latches on, then that's wonderful. She probably won't suck for long but enough to give you an idea of what it feels like.

Don't be surprised if you feel strong contraction-like pains. Breastfeeding stimulates your uterus to contract, to go back to it's pre-pregnancy size, which is sometimes what causes these after-pains. You may feel these pains every time you feed for the first few weeks, but then they should stop. However, not everyone feels them, and they are often less painful for first babies.

If your baby doesn't show any interest in feeding straight away, don't worry. She might be sleepy to begin with, after the tiring experience of labour, or she might be very alert and more interested in looking at the world around her. Enjoy holding her and looking at her – the skin-to-skin contact alone is enough to stimulate your milk supply. You can try offering her your breast again later.

TOP TIP

To remember which breast to start feeding on, wear a wrist band or ring and move it from side to side as appropriate. If you need to feed from your left breast next time, wear your wrist band on your left hand. It's a great visual reminder.

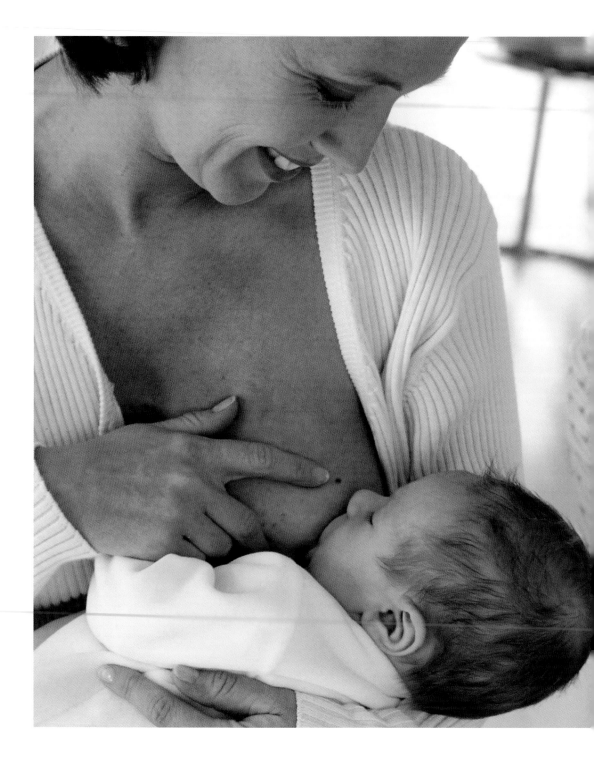

Chapter 3

BREASTFEEDING Keep going

It takes time for you and your baby to get to know each other. Even if this isn't your first baby, there's so much to learn and it's a new experience for both of you. It's hard to know what to expect; you may be surprised by how much time is spent feeding. Your emotions may be unpredictable, too. Some days you may feel full of energy, self-confident and experience a sense of achievement when your baby is feeding well and everything is going right. Other days you may feel down if your baby seems unsettled and you haven't been able to get anything done except feed. You may feel so tired that everything seems to be a blur. But the important thing is to keep going.

Practise makes perfect

Gradually, as your baby grows and you become more practised at breastfeeding, things will get easier. You will both start to know what you're doing! A routine may start to emerge, and you will start to get more sleep at night. While some women find that breastfeeding comes very easily to them, others may find it takes a bit longer before they feel fully confident. As a rough guide, health professionals advise that it takes six weeks to properly establish breastfeeding and to physically adapt to the supply and demand of milk-producing. It is recommended that you breastfeed exclusively for this period of time before you try another method of feeding. Keep persevering and before you know it you'll be an expert breastfeeder.

The early days

For the first few days and weeks your baby needs to feed little and often, roughly every 2– 3 hours, or 8– 12 times in 24 hours. This is because her tummy is so small it gets full very quickly and empties very quickly. Feeding frequently is also important to help establish your milk supply *(see page 9)*.

You may find that your newborn baby is very sleepy for the first few days and not interested in feeding. If this is the case, you will need to wake her up. Try undressing her and having skin-to-skin contact with her to help wake her up. Gently blowing on her face should keep her awake if she keeps on falling asleep while you're feeding her.

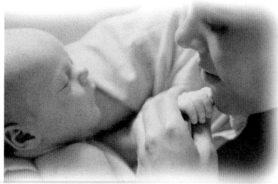

The sleepy period usually only lasts a few days. If your baby is really lethargic and disinterested and shows no periods of being alert, talk to your midwife.

In the hospital: if this is your first baby, the chances are that the birth was in hospital and that this is where you are likely to stay for the first day.

Whether you are in hospital for only a few hours or a few days, do take advantage of all the experienced staff there; ask them for help and advice on feeding your baby or any other issues. No question is too silly or unimportant – the staff will be happy to provide support and reassurance.

Maternity wards often have a nursing room where you can feed your baby and possibly meet other mums who are either learning to breastfeed for the first time or who have the benefit of experience. This can be useful.

TOP TIP
Wrapping your baby securely in swaddling blankets to stop her from waving her arms about can help make feeding easier.

Going home: leaving the hospital and going home is an exciting day, but it can be a bit daunting, too. Whether your home is full of family and friends to support you, or whether you are on your own, it's important to remember that your community midwife and/or health visitor is there to give support and advice. They will visit you to make sure that you and your baby are doing well and will answer any feeding questions you may have.

The first 12 weeks

TOP TIP
However much you want to show your new baby off, or how much your relatives and friends want to see the new member of the family, try to limit the number of visitors in the first few weeks. You need this time just to think about your baby and feeding her, rather than worrying about cleaning the house or making cups of tea and coffee.

After the first few days, your baby will start demanding food herself. How often she wants to be fed and for how long is different for each baby. Some babies will want to feed every hour, but will get a full feed after only 10 minutes at the breast. Other babies may last as long as four hours between feeds, but will spend 40–50 minutes feeding. It will vary from day to day and feed to feed. Be led by your baby. She will eat as much as she needs to and when she's had enough she will stop sucking and come off the breast herself.

Feeding your baby on demand rather than by the clock ensures that you will be meeting all her nutritional needs and that you will make the correct amount of milk. A generation or so ago, it was popular for babies to be fed on a strict timetable basis. Mothers were encouraged to feed their babies for only 20 minutes every four hours, whether or not the baby seemed to be satisfied by this. Although for some babies and mothers this worked, today the importance of baby-led feeding is generally accepted. Your baby knows when she is hungry and your body will respond by producing the required amount of milk. If your baby isn't allowed to feed when she's hungry, but only when you let her feed, then your body won't necessarily be producing the right amount of milk.

A pattern emerges: demand or baby-led feeding can mean that you will spend a lot of your day feeding, particularly in the early days, and you may wonder whether you will ever get any routine back in your life. It may take time, but gradually a pattern will emerge when your baby wants to feed. With some babies, a pattern emerges after only a few weeks, with others it may take a few months but as your baby grows and as you both get better at feeding you will find the time between feeds gradually gets longer and the times that she wants to feed become more regular. You will come to know your baby better, and her behaviour will start to become more predictable.

Growth spurts: just as you think you have established a regular feeding pattern, your baby may suddenly start wanting to feed more frequently because she is having a growth spurt. This commonly happens at 10 days, six weeks and three months, but it varies with each baby. No one knows exactly why these growth spurts occur, but they are believed to be linked to important developmental changes.

4–6 months

Your baby will have changed a lot in the first three months. She is no longer 'newborn', although she still depends on you completely for everything she needs. She will be taking an interest in the world around her, smiling as she recognises you and other members of her family, and generally being more active. Her feeding requirements will have changed by now, too. As she becomes more active, she will be getting hungrier and need to drink more milk.

If your baby is emptying both breasts at every feed, so that she is feeding well and not snacking too much in between, she should be having roughly five feeds a day. This will provide her with around 175ml (6fl oz) of milk at each feed, which should mean that she can sleep through the night without needing a feed.

Current government guidelines state that babies should not start solids until they are six months old because breast and formula milk provide all the required nutrients until then. However, all babies are different and some may seem to need to start solids earlier than this. You should consult your health visitor or GP if you feel this might be the case.

When your baby is six months old you can start to introduce solids into her diet, but very gradually. Your baby should still be getting the same number of milk feeds as before, i.e. five feeds during the day with 3–4 hours between each feed. By now both breasts will be producing roughly 250ml (8fl oz) of milk at every feed.

7–9 months

By the time your baby is seven months old, she should be eating quite a range of different solid foods, but she will still be drinking about 600ml (20fl oz) of milk a day. She may have dropped a feed so that she is only getting milk feeds three or four times during the day at roughly breakfast time, mid-morning or mid-afternoon and bedtime. Although your baby will be much more independent now and want to feed herself with solid food, the milk feeds are still an important time when you can be together and enjoy each other's close contact.

How to check if your baby is getting enough milk

Because you can't see how much milk your baby is drinking, it is easy to worry about whether she's getting enough, especially if she wants to feed all the time or she doesn't seem satisfied after a feed. There are two main indicators that your baby is getting enough milk:

Weight gain: if your baby puts on weight steadily you will know she is feeding properly. Having said this, it's usual for a baby to lose up to 10 per cent of her birth weight within the first week of life. After that, however, she should start to gain weight at a rate of about 30g (1oz) per day. By the time she is two weeks old she should have regained her birth weight; by six months she should have doubled her birth weight. After this, weight gain gradually slows down. You can get your baby weighed at your local clinic, usually every week, to check that she is gaining weight satisfactorily. Your health visitor will advise you if you have any concerns.

Wet nappies: checking your baby's nappies is another good way of judging whether she is getting enough milk. For the first couple of days she will excrete a dark sticky substance called meconium that built up in her intestines while she was in the womb. To begin with she won't wet her nappies very often, but after the first few days your baby should be wetting around 6–8 nappies a day. From around the fifth day she will do about two poos a day, which by now should be soft and a mustard yellow colour. Your baby's urine should be a pale colour and shouldn't smell.

Other signs that your baby is getting enough milk include:

● She takes the breast happily and stays latched on until she's finished.

● Your breasts feel softer after feeds.

● She seems contented after feeds.

How to recognise when your baby is hungry

Your baby will give you lots of signs that she's hungry and as you get to know her these will become clearer to you. Here are some signs to look out for:

- Putting her hand in her mouth and sucking her fingers or her fist.

- Rooting for your breast by turning her head towards you and looking for your nipple.

- Becoming agitated, kicking her legs and waving her arms around.

- Making noises.

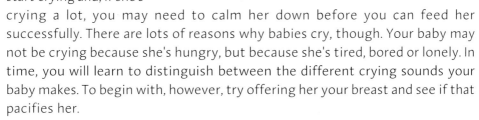

If you don't take any notice of these signals, sooner or later your baby will start crying and, if she's crying a lot, you may need to calm her down before you can feed her successfully. There are lots of reasons why babies cry, though. Your baby may not be crying because she's hungry, but because she's tired, bored or lonely. In time, you will learn to distinguish between the different crying sounds your baby makes. To begin with, however, try offering her your breast and see if that pacifies her.

Feeding your baby at night

In the beginning you will be feeding your baby at the same intervals throughout the night as you do during the day. Your baby needs to be fed at night because she can only last a few hours between feeds, and the comfort and closeness of being with you is important to her. It will be a while before your baby can sleep through the night.

Feeding your baby at night can be a very special time when everything is quiet and there's nothing to distract you. For this reason you may not mind having a broken sleep. But if your baby is waking up frequently for a feed, or seems to have muddled up night and day, sleeping for long periods during the day but staying awake at night, you will feel exhausted the next day and may wonder whether you'll ever have a decent night's sleep again.

Here are some suggestions for things you can do from an early age to encourage your baby to go back to sleep quickly after a feed at night so you can get some sleep too:

- During the day, try not to let your baby sleep for too long between feeds.

- Give your baby a bedtime routine. Bath her, change her and then feed her in a darkened room before putting her down to sleep. It's helpful if she's still a little awake when you put her down, so that she learns how to go to sleep alone.

- When she wakes in the night, keep the lighting and your voice low and make the feed as boring as possible. Try not to chat to her too much or distract her.

- Make sure she is properly winded before putting her back down again.

- Don't change her nappy unless you need to to avoid distracting her.

You may also find it helpful to wake your baby and feed her just before you go to bed so you get a few hours' sleep at least before she wakes again for another feed.

Sharing a bed with your baby

You may find that night-time feeding is a lot easier if your baby sleeps in bed with you. As it is easy to fall asleep while breastfeeding, especially when lying down, there are some important points to consider before taking your baby into bed with you. Falling asleep with your baby is dangerous if you:

- or any other person in the bed is a smoker, even if you never smoke in bed;

- have drunk alcohol;

- have taken any drug (legal or illegal) which could make you extra sleepy;

- have any illness or condition which affects your awareness of your baby;

- are otherwise unusually tired to a point where you would find it difficult to respond to your baby.

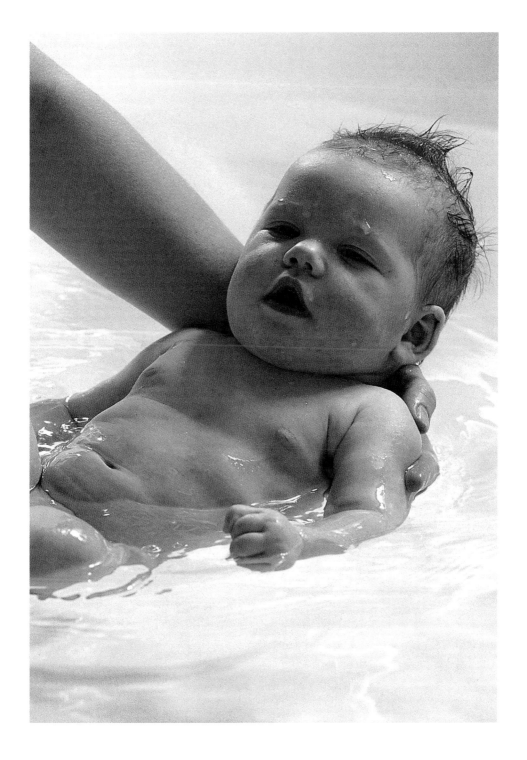

It's also not a good idea to sleep with any sibling toddlers and you must *never* sleep with your baby on a sofa or armchair.

The advantages are:

- You don't have to get out of bed to feed her.

- You can doze while your baby feeds and settles back to sleep.

- She may get back to sleep more quickly and easily with the security of having you next to her.

- Sleeping next to your baby can promote a feeling of emotional closeness. Some studies claim that babies who sleep in the same bed sleep for longer periods during the night.

The disadvantages are:

- You may worry unnecessarily about rolling on top of your baby and so sleep less well.

- If your baby is used to falling asleep next to you, it may make it more difficult for her to go to sleep at night without you.

- Intimacy in bed between you and your partner is more difficult.

Expressing breast milk

After you have established breastfeeding, you may find that expressing your milk helps you to keep on going. It is a technique that involves squeezing milk out of your breasts, either manually or with a pump, so that it can be stored in bottles and given to your baby later. It may sound unappealing, but expressing milk can actually be very useful for a number of reasons:

TOP TIP
Have a high-energy snack around teatime. This is the time you often feel most tired, which can affect your milk supply.

- It allows someone else to feed your baby. If you need to go back to work, or you are unwell and unable to feed your baby, or you want to go out for an evening, you can do this while your baby still benefits from receiving your milk.

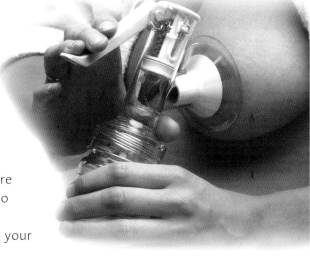

● It means your partner can give your baby a night-time feed occasionally so that you can have some sleep. This will also help him feel more involved in your baby's care.

● Premature or special-care babies who are unable to feed directly from your breast can benefit from your breast milk.

● It can stimulate your milk supply and so help to prolong breastfeeding.

● It should help relieve swollen or engorged breasts.

Expressing by hand: although this is the most economical way of expressing your milk, it can take a long time to do and will probably require quite a lot of practise. It's usually easier to do it in the morning when you have a full milk supply. You might find it easier if you express in a warm bath or shower, or with your baby near to you.

1. Make sure your hands are clean before you start.

2. Sit at a table with a sterilised bowl or container under your breast.

3. Hold your breast in a C-hold, placing your thumb at the top edge of the areola (the dark skin around your nipple) and using the rest of your hand to cup your breast underneath.

4. Carefully squeeze your finger and thumb together and pull forward.

5. Continue doing this in a rhythmic way until the milk flows. It may take a while

TOP TIP
Write the date on the bottle or bag of expressed milk before storing it so you know how old it is.

for the milk to appear, and at first you may not produce very much milk, but it's worth persevering. With practise you should be able to do it.

If you are planning to express on a regular basis, electric or manual breast pumps are often faster and more efficient. They are more expensive, but it is possible to hire pumps from the hospital or organisations such as the National Childbirth Trust *(see page 70)*. Breast pumps work by suction. With an electric pump, a cup is placed over your breast, and when the machine is turned on it mechanically creates a suction to release your milk into a container. With a manual pump, the suction is created by a squeeze mechanism *(see page 37)*. On average it takes 15–30 minutes to pump both breasts with an electric pump and 30–45 minutes with a manual pump.

HOW TO STORE BREAST MILK

The best way to store breast milk is in a sterilised plastic feeding bottle, which has a secure top. You can also buy plastic bags made especially for storing milk. Breast milk can be stored in a fridge running below 10°C for up to three days or you can keep it in the freezer at -18°C or lower for up to six months. Never use a microwave to warm up bottled breast milk because the microwaves kill all the beneficial nutrients.

Common concerns

Can I combine breastfeeding with using a bottle for feeding my baby expressed milk?

Yes, combined or mixed feeding can work well for some mothers. However, it is best to wait until after your baby is six weeks old so that she has got really used to breastfeeding before you introduce something new. Sucking from a bottle requires a different technique to sucking a breast and it's important that your baby doesn't get 'nipple confusion', which is more likely to happen if you introduce a bottle too early.

You may find that your baby doesn't want to accept a bottle immediately, preferring your breast. You will need to be patient as it may take a few days of offering her the bottle at different times before she will accept it. Here are some tips for helping your baby to take a bottle:

- Get someone else to offer her the bottle so she's not expecting to be breastfed.

- If you are giving her the bottle, hold her away from your breast, in a different position from the one you would normally feed her in.

- Try feeding her in between her normal feed time so that she's not too desperately hungry for your breast or too full to bother.

- Try different types of teat.

How long should I Breastfeed for?

The basic answer is that you should breastfeed for as long as both you and your baby want to. Some women breastfeed for only a few weeks, others may breastfeed for as long as a year, or more. The World Health Organization recommends breastfeeding exclusively for the first six months and then continuing while you introduce solid foods, but this is not necessarily possible or desirable for everyone. Even if you have only been able to breastfeed your baby for a few weeks, you will have given her a good start in life.

TOP TIP
Consider buying or borrowing a double electric breast pump. You will express your milk in half the time which is especially handy with twins or more!

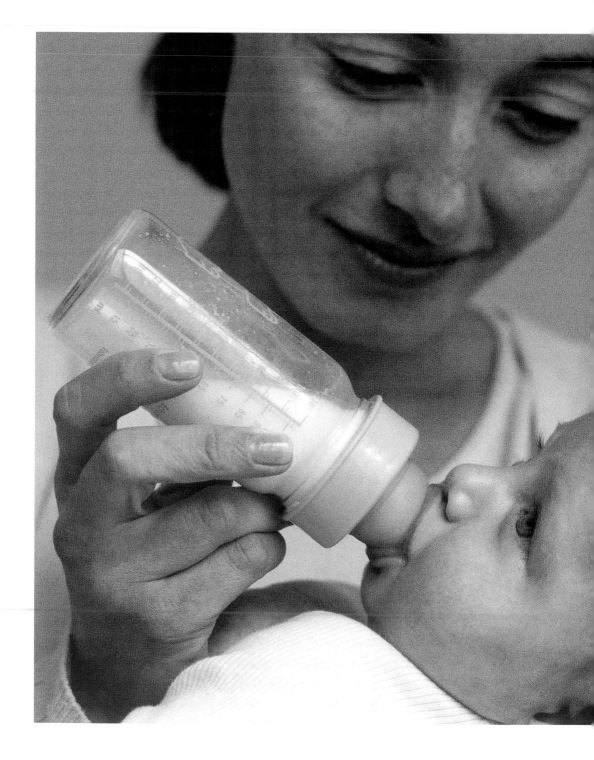

Chapter 4

BOTTLE-FEEDING What you need to know

There may be many reasons why you have decided to bottle-feed your baby formula milk, ranging from wanting to share the feeding of your baby with your partner and family, to finding breastfeeding too difficult and painful. Whether you have decided to bottle-feed your baby from birth or whether you are switching to bottle-feeding from breastfeeding, you can be assured that your baby will be getting all the essential nutrients she needs to grow and develop healthily.

A healthy start

Bottle-feeding your baby can be a deeply warm, loving and bonding experience just like breastfeeding. Whatever your reasons for choosing to bottle-feed, the important thing is to feel confident in your chosen method. There is a lot of pressure on mothers to breastfeed and this can make women who bottle-feed feel guilty and unhappy. Remember that there are benefits to bottle-feeding, too, and that your baby is being given a perfectly healthy start to her life. In the end, the best method of feeding your baby is the one that works for the two of you. A relaxed and contented mother and baby is what is most important.

What is formula milk?

Infant formula milk is the only alternative to breast milk. It either comes in powder form, which you reconstitute by adding boiled water, or ready-made in cartons – this latter option is the more expensive.

There are different types of formula milk available, but most are made from cows' milk with ingredients added to make them suitable and digestible for a baby. For example, unsaturated vegetable oils are added to give formula milk the right fat content. Sugars are also added, and salts are reduced. However, since breast milk is always changing, the exact chemical make-up is impossible to reproduce.

The main types of formula for babies under six months are:

Whey-based formula: whey is a type of milk protein that is most easily absorbed by babies and the most similar to breast milk. This type of formula can be given to babies from birth.

Casein-based formula: casein is another type of milk protein but one that is less easily absorbed by babies. This type of formula is said to satisfy more hungry babies because the casein is not so digestible so your baby feels full for longer. It is suitable to give from birth.

TOP TIP
Boiled water is needed to make up a formula feed, so a fast and efficient kettle that can hold quite a lot of water is a real benefit.

Specialist formula: specialist formula milk is prescribed by GPs for babies who can't tolerate cows' milk formula.

Ordinary cows' milk, goats' milk, condensed milk, dried milk, evaporated milk or any other type of milk should never be given to a baby under 12 months old. If you are unsure about what type of formula to give your baby or have any other concerns about bottle-feeding, ask your midwife or health visitor for advice.

TOP TIP
Powdered formula milk is not sterile so to avoid any risk of infection, the bottles of formula must only be made up as they are needed, never prepared in advance.

Bottles and teats
There are a huge number of bottle-feeding accessories available in the shops designed to make bottle-feeding easier. Listed below are some essential items:

Bottles: these come in two sizes and different shapes. The smaller size, which takes 113ml (4fl oz), is designed for the newborn baby. The larger size takes up to 255ml (9fl oz), which a bigger baby will take. However, there is no reason why you can't feed your newborn baby the small amount of milk she needs from a larger bottle.

Teats: again you will find a wide variety of teats in different shapes and sizes. Some claim to reduce the likelihood of colic by restricting the amount of air that is swallowed; others claim to be the most orthodontic friendly. The teats have different-sized holes to vary the rate at which the milk comes out. A newborn baby will need a slow-flowing teat. As your baby grows, try out the faster-flowing teats to satisfy her hunger more quickly.

Bottle and teat brushes: cleaning bottles and teats properly is very important. Specially designed brushes will make the job a lot easier.

Sterilising
Because small babies are particularly vulnerable to getting infections, all the equipment you use to feed your baby, including the bottles, teats, caps and even the knife you use to level off the formula powder, must be sterilised to kill off any bacteria.

There are several methods of sterilising:

Cold water and sterilising tablets: this is an economical method, although time-consuming. All the equipment is placed in a sterilising unit (plastic bucket) to which cold water is added together with a chemical sterilising solution or tablets. It takes 30 minutes for the equipment to be sterilised and then everything needs to be rinsed carefully with cooled boiled water.

Steamers: electric and microwave steamers are available. They are very simple and quick to use, although they are more expensive to buy. You put the bottles and other equipment into the steamer and several minutes later (exact time depends on the appliance) enough steam has been created to sterilise your equipment.

Boiling water: put everything that needs to be sterilised in a large pan of boiling water and boil for 10 minutes. You need to make sure that everything is completely submerged. Keep the pan covered until the equipment is needed. This is the most economical way to sterilise equipment, but not always convenient and the regular boiling tends to wear out the teats more quickly than other methods.

Other bottle-feeding accessories

Here are some things that aren't essential for feeding but which you may find helpful:

Bottle warmer: most babies prefer to drink warm milk rather than milk that has come straight from the fridge. An electric bottle warmer is useful for warming up pre-boiled cooled water or cartons of ready-made formula milk quickly, for instance when you are feeding at night.

Milk powder dispenser: to help you make up your formula feeds when you are out and about these little units carry pre-measured doses of milk powder in separate compartments. When you're ready to feed, you just open the spout and pour the powder into the bottle of pre-boiled cooled water.

How to prepare a feed

Before you make up your baby's feed, the bottles need to have been washed in hot soapy water and then sterilised.

You will find directions on the tin for how to make up the formula, including how many scoops of powder you will need for the weight/age of your baby. Remember that powdered infant formula is not sterile so to avoid any risk of infection you must only prepare each feed as it is needed.

It's really important to make sure that good hygiene practices are followed when preparing the feeds. Here are the basic steps and information:

1. Clean the surface where you will be preparing the feeds and wash your hands.

2. Boil fresh tap water in a kettle or pan. Water that has been boiled repeatedly in a kettle should not be used because it will have too much sodium. Mineral water should not be used either because it is subject to less health regulation than ordinary tap water and may contain higher concentrations of minerals than is safe for your baby.

3. Leave the boiled water to cool, but not for more than half an hour. Official guidelines state that the water should not be less than 70ºC (158ºF) when you add the formula.

4. Pour the required amount of water into the sterilised bottles and add the precise amount of formula following the directions on the tin. The usual guideline is one level scoop of formula per 28ml (1fl oz) of water. It's very important to add the powder to the water and not the other way round so that you ensure you get the right quantity. If you add too much or too little powder, your baby could become ill. Always use a sterilised knife to level off each scoop.

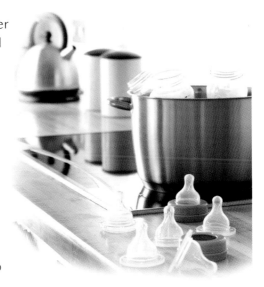

5. Fit the teat and cap back on the bottle and shake it to mix up the contents.

6. It should be lukewarm – just above body temperature. Test it out by shaking a few drops onto the inside of your wrist. If necessary, cool it down by holding it in a jug of cold water or under a running tap.

7. Once your baby has drunk from a bottle, throw away any milk that has not been used within two hours.

STORING BOTTLED MILK

In the past, it was common to make up all the bottles your baby needed for the day in one go. However, in November 2005 the Department of Health changed its advice and now recommends that a fresh bottle is made up for each feed. This is because formula milk is not sterile and there is a small risk of contamination from micro-organisms if made up formula is kept. If you need to prepare bottles in advance, the advice is to store freshly boiled water in bottles which you can warm up when you need them and then add the formula milk at the last minute.

How to bottle-feed your baby

Bottle-feeding your baby can be a wonderful bonding experience. Most babies take to it easily so you can peacefully enjoy the experience without worrying whether or not the feeding is going well.

1. Find a comfortable, quiet place to feed your baby. A chair that supports your back and your arm while you are holding your baby is ideal.

2. Hold your baby with her head in the crook of your arm and bring her in close to you. This will make her feel safe, secure and relaxed, which will help her to feed. She should be held so that her head is higher than her stomach to help digestion and so that her back is straight and not rounded. This will help prevent too much air being swallowed.

3. Tilt the bottle so that the teat fills with milk and not air and keep it tilted all the time you are feeding her. Swallowing too much air while she is sucking will not only make her very windy, which can be uncomfortable, but is also thought to be a contributing factor to colic.

4. Use the time while your baby is feeding to bond with her. She will probably look into your eyes and study your face. Smile, sing or talk softly to her and tell her how beautiful she is. She won't understand the words, but she will understand the love behind them. Let her take as much time as she likes to feed. She may fall asleep for a little in the middle of the feed and then wake shortly after wanting to finish the feed.

5. Your baby may need winding *(see page 22–23)* in the middle of the feed, at the end of the feed, or both. Don't stop her in the middle of a feed unnecessarily, though, because she will get very frustrated! It's a good idea to have a muslin cloth to hand because she will probably 'sick up' (posset) or regurgitate some of the milk.

The first time you feed your baby

TOP TIP
If the teat flattens so your baby can't get any milk, gently remove the bottle from your baby's mouth to release the vacuum.

If you have decided to bottle-feed your baby from birth, try giving her a bottle as soon as you are ready. Your midwife will be able to help you and may prepare the first few feeds so that you can concentrate on giving the bottle. She may give you a choice of brands, but unless you have a strong preference there is very little to choose between them. The midwife can also show your partner how to prepare the feeds. Alternatively the hospital may provide you with bottles of ready-made formula with disposable

BREAST DISCOMFORT

For the first few days after giving birth you may feel some breast discomfort because they will have produced milk ready to feed, and it will take time for them to go back to normal. You may find that your breasts will leak some milk, so it's helpful to have a few breast pads handy to wear inside your bra to absorb the milk.

teats. When you leave hospital try to carry on using the same brand of formula that your baby has been having.

During the early days, you and your baby will be getting to know each other. It may help get things off to a good start if you can have skin-to-skin contact while you are feeding her.

How much to feed your baby and how often

When bottle-feeding, unlike breastfeeding, you can tell exactly how much milk your baby is taking. This can be very reassuring.

The advice for how much to feed your newborn baby is the same as breastfed babies. Be led by your baby, feed her as often as she asks for it and don't worry how often she wants feeding. In the early days, she will need to be fed little and often, possibly only 50ml (2fl oz) every one or two hours.

By the time she is two or three weeks old, your baby may be able to go for longer between feeds and she will probably be taking around 85ml (3fl oz) every 2–3 hours.

A feeding pattern will emerge quite soon with your bottle-fed baby. If she is feeding roughly every three hours, she will be taking 6–8 feeds a day. The amount she drinks will steadily increase from 85–113ml (3–4fl oz) at one month old to as much as 198–227ml (7–8fl oz) by the time she is four months old when she will probably have settled into a pattern of five feeds a day.

There are rough guidelines to feeding amounts and frequency on the tins of formula milk, but it's important to remember they are only guidelines and that every baby is different. If your baby doesn't want to finish her bottle, she will probably take herself off the teat or stop sucking. If she is still hungry at the end of a feed and wants more milk than you've given her, she

TOP TIP

Never prop up a bottle and leave your baby to feed herself as she could choke.

will cry. It's a good idea to make up bottles with slightly more milk than she usually drinks so that she can leave a little if she doesn't want it, but still be satisfied if her appetite increases.

Night-time feeds

Your formula-fed baby will need feeding during the night at first, probably before you go to bed at around 11pm, then at around 2am and then in the early morning at around 6am. One of the benefits of bottle-feeding, of course, is that the night-time feeds can be shared with your partner, so that you are able to get some sleep. These feeds will be a lot easier if you have the bottles of cooled boiled water prepared before you go to bed so that you just need to add the milk powder. Having a bottle warmer next to your bed will make it easy for you to heat the bottle with the minimum disturbance. Don't forget to check the temperature first by shaking a few drops onto your wrist.

By the time your baby is two months old she may well have dropped the feed in the middle of the night so that she is getting (and so are you!) a seven- or eight- hour stretch of uninterrupted sleep.

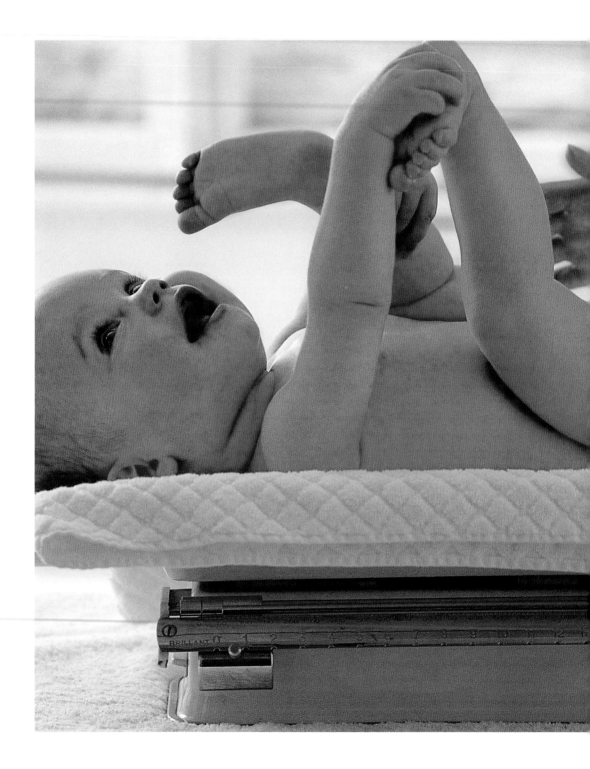

Chapter 5

COMMON FEEDING CONCERNS
How to overcome them

However easy and enjoyable you find feeding, there may be times when things don't happen as they're meant to, or problems arise which cause worry and concern. Early problems with breastfeeding, in particular, are common and you may find feeding painful at times or have problems with your milk supply. Other concerns you may have might include how to feed your baby when you are away from home or what to do if you have given birth to more than one baby. If you have a baby with special needs you may also have specific feeding concerns.

Common concerns

There is often a simple remedy to common feeding concerns and the earlier you deal with a problem the more effective the remedy and the least disruptive and upsetting the situation will be for you and your baby. Being aware of what problems might arise may also help you to avoid them altogether.

Breastfeeding problems

Perhaps the most common concern that breastfeeding mothers have is what to do when breastfeeding causes pain and discomfort. The answer to this depends on the reason why breastfeeding hurts. Often it is because your baby isn't latched on to your nipple properly *(see pages 20–21)* which can cause sore, cracked nipples and blisters. Your health visitor, midwife or breastfeeding supporter can help resolve this problem by checking how your baby is latching on. But there are other problems which can occur with breastfeeding. The most common of these are listed below together with suggestions for what to do.

Engorgement: this is when your breasts become hugely swollen and feel very uncomfortable and hard. This usually happens between the third and fifth day after your baby is born, when your mature milk comes in. It can also happen when you stop breastfeeding if you do so too abruptly – the weaning process needs to happen gradually.

What to do: although it may be painful, you need to keep on feeding your baby as much as possible to reduce the swelling. Your breasts should start to feel better within a couple of days. You can take paracetamol or ibuprofen painkillers without harming your baby. Check your baby is latching on properly *(see pages 20–21)*. If your breasts have got so large that your nipples have flattened, try expressing some milk to relieve the swelling. A popular remedy which has been used successfully for centuries to reduce the swelling is to apply refrigerated cabbage leaves to your breasts! Put the leaves inside your bra, making sure you have covered your breasts completely, and leave for up to half an hour or whenever the leaves have wilted. Repeat as necessary until the swelling has gone down.

Blocked milk ducts: your milk ducts can become blocked – forming a small painful lump in your breast and causing inflammation – if your baby doesn't completely empty your breast of milk when she feeds.

What to do: this shouldn't happen if you are feeding often and making sure that your baby finishes one breast before starting another. Vary your feeding positions *(see pages 18– 20)* so that your baby is more able to remove the milk from all of your milk ducts. Avoid wearing anything too tight around your breasts, including an underwired bra. Massage your breast as you feed your baby to help unblock the duct. Also try applying a warm flannel or cloth to your breast for a few minutes before you feed.

Mastitis: if a blocked duct becomes infected it can lead to mastitis which is sometimes extremely painful. This bacterial infection can cause your breasts to become swollen, red and lumpy and is accompanied by flu-like symptoms and a high temperature. Occasionally mastitis can lead to an abscess, which is a more severe form of infection where pus forms in your breast. This will require urgent medical attention.

TOP TIP
Don't abandon breastfeeding if you are suffering from mastitis. You may feel ill and discouraged but continuing to breastfeed is the quickest way to get better – and it won't hurt your baby.

What to do: Taking ibuprofen reduces the inflammation, relieves pain and reduces temperature. Take 400mg three times a day after food. Paracetamol also relieves pain and reduces temperature but has no anti-inflammatory action. Take two 500mg tablets four times a day. Antibiotics may be needed if mastitis is due to a bacterial infection. To help avoid developing mastitis, follow the advice for blocked milk ducts *(see page 52)*.

Thrush: this is a fungal infection that can affect both mother and baby. It is also known as candida. You may notice white spots on your breasts and in your baby's mouth, which makes feeding uncomfortable. Your baby may also get a nasty case of nappy rash, and you may feel sharp shooting pains deep in your breasts, which may also feel itchy. It often appears after a course of antibiotics and can spread from mother to baby via breastfeeding.

What to do: your doctor will prescribe an antifungal cream for both of you, which should clear up the problem quickly. You do not need to give up breastfeeding. However, it is important that you are both treated at the same time to prevent you from re-infecting each other. There are a number of things you can do at home which should ensure that thrush doesn't recur:

● The infection thrives in damp, warm places so change your nursing pads after every feed and change your baby's nappy frequently.

● Wash your hands before and after each feed.

● Use a separate towel for each person in the family.

● Eat 145ml (5fl oz) of live yoghurt a day – it contains fungus-destroying probiotics.

● Ask your partner to be tested because the infection can easily be transmitted.

Teeth: A common concern for many mothers is how to breastfeed a baby with teeth. Will she bite? And, if so, how do you stop her? The average age for a baby to start teething is six months. Although some mothers will have stopped breastfeeding by then and may have weaned their baby onto solids and cup-feeding, many mothers are still breastfeeding. Lots of babies with teeth don't ever bite their mothers – but there are some that do. If this happens once, you want to make sure it doesn't happen again!

What to do: if your baby is teething she may be suffering from sore gums and will chew on everything in sight. In the hope that she doesn't chew you, try giving her a teething toy to chew on before or after you feed her. If this doesn't work, however, and your baby does bite you, she needs to get the firm message not to do it again. If you react to her bite with a loud noise (for example, a scream), this may shock her into not doing it again. However, it could make her curious to see if she gets the same reaction a second time. Stop feeding her at the same time as saying 'No' firmly. You can finish the feed by offering her water or juice in a baby cup and try breastfeeding again later.

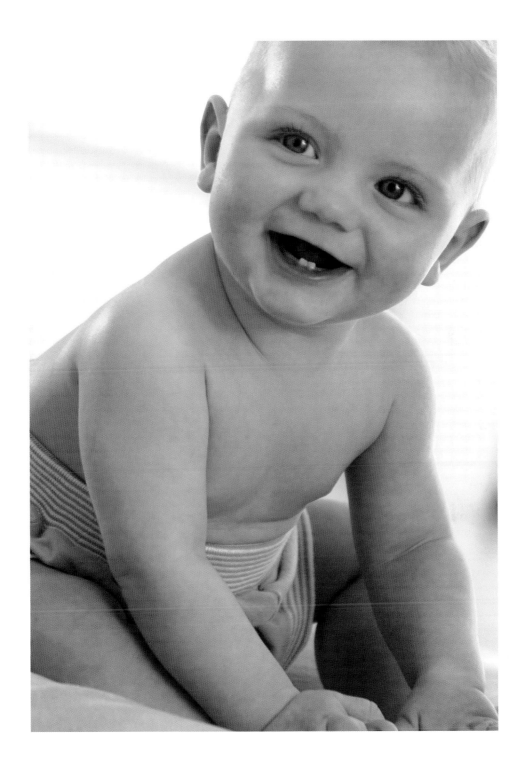

Weight

How much your baby weighs will probably be something you think about a lot and possibly worry about while your baby is small, as her weight is an indication of how well she is feeding and thriving. However, try not to be too concerned about this. In the early days your midwife will weigh your baby as often as necessary when she makes her home visits. After that, getting your baby weighed at the baby clinic every few weeks should be quite enough.

Underfed babies: if your baby is not gaining weight sufficiently, you will need to find out the reason why. If she is breastfed, the most common reason is that she isn't latching on well *(see pages 20–21)*. Another possibility is that she may have a *tongue tie*, although this is not commonly seen. When a baby is tongue-tied the stringy tissue, or frenulum, that connects the tongue to the bottom of the mouth is too short and tight. This prevents your baby sticking her tongue out far enough, and may affect her ability to suck properly.

What to do: if you breastfeed, first ask your midwife or health visitor to check your baby's positioning as she latches on. If she is latching on correctly she should be able to take as much milk as she needs to grow. If, however, she is tongue-tied, her frenulum may need to be snipped – a procedure that takes seconds and doesn't hurt the baby at all – so that the tongue can move properly. This should make breastfeeding easier and reduce the possibility of speech problems later in life.

Overfed babies

Overfeeding can be a problem with bottle-fed babies. If a baby finishes her bottle quickly and then cries at the end, it is common to assume she is still hungry and give her more formula. In fact she may be crying, not from hunger, but because she wants to carry on sucking. Quite quickly a pattern of overfeeding can develop and your baby could put on more weight than is good for her.

TOP TIP
If your baby is not gaining sufficient weight, it may be that she is not getting enough of the rich hind milk, in which case you need to speak to your health visitor, midwife or breastfeeding supporter to find out why.

What to do: this problem should be

discussed with your health visitor, but can easily be remedied by spacing your baby's feeds appropriately and ensuring she is given the right amount of formula in each feed. When a bottle-fed baby has fed but still wants to suck, giving her a dummy to replace the bottle might help.

More than one baby

If you have given birth to twins, or more, you may be particularly worried about how you will be able to feed them. It is perfectly possible to breastfeed them all if you want to, because your body will respond to their feeding demands and produce enough milk. Even more so than with one baby, however, you will need to make sure you get as much support as you can from your partner, family and friends.

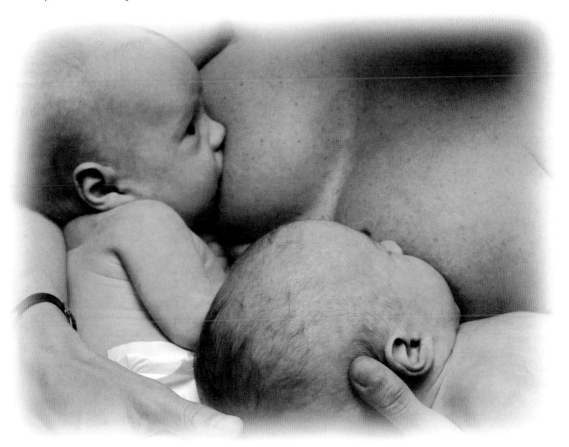

PREMATURE BABIES

If your baby is born prematurely, your breasts will produce a special milk called pre-term milk, which has a high fat content and extra nutrients to help your baby grow and develop. Depending on how early your baby is born, you might be able to breastfeed her yourself but if she weighs less than 1.5kg (3lb 5oz) or is born before 29 weeks, she will not be able to suck properly. If this is the case, you will need to use a breast pump *(see pages 13, 37–38)* as soon as possible after your baby is born so that she can be given your milk through a tube that goes through her mouth and into her stomach.

If you decide to breastfeed your babies, you will need to decide whether you want to feed your babies one at a time or two at a time. It may help to start off feeding them separately, until you get the hang of it. This is easier if your babies want to be fed at different times. If two babies are hungry at the same time, you will need someone to help you with looking after the waiting baby. Make sure that your babies take it in turns to wait. Feeding your babies separately, while giving you lots of practise, also means that almost all of your time will be spent feeding.

If you are breastfeeding two babies at the same time, you will need pillows or cushions to support them on either side of you and to raise them to the right height for feeding. One advantage of feeding them together is that they will probably want to sleep at the same time too, giving you time to sleep as well. Tiredness is one of the biggest problems you will face when feeding more than one baby.

You only have two breasts so if you have more than two babies, one is definitely going to have to wait – unless you express milk so that the other baby/babies can be given a bottle of your milk by another person.

If you are bottle-feeding your babies, it is probably easier to feed them one at a time, although some mothers put their babies in their car seats to feed them together. Remember that you should never prop up a bottle and leave your baby to feed herself as she could choke.

Feeding out and about

In some ways, breastfeeding is the perfect way to feed your baby when you're away from home. You don't need to worry about packing up lots of equipment, or how long you're going to be out for; so long as you are with your baby, you can feed her wherever and whenever you like. Sadly, many women are concerned about breastfeeding in public perhaps because while public opinion is generally more accepting of this now, it is still the case that breastfeeding in public is not a legal right in England, as it is in Scotland.

TOP TIP

If you are carrying your baby in a babysling with her facing towards you it is possible to breastfeed your baby while you are walking about without exposing anything and without anyone noticing.

Don't be put off, though. Most people are very understanding about the need to feed your child and once you are practised at breastfeeding and can feed discreetly, the chances are that no one will even notice. It's easier if you wear a front-opening top so that you don't have to expose too much of yourself! If

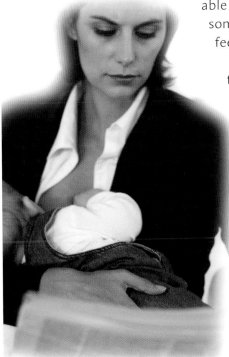

you still find it difficult, you will probably be able to find a breastfeeding room or somewhere equally quiet so that you can feed in private.

If you are bottle-feeding, you will need to be organised and plan ahead if you are going to be away from home for any length of time with your baby. The simplest thing to do is to take cartons of ready-made formula which can be used instantly. Alternatively you will need to take the formula powder separately and add measured amounts to the bottles of cooled boiled water when you are ready to feed. Many restaurants and cafes are happy to warm up a baby bottle if you ask them.

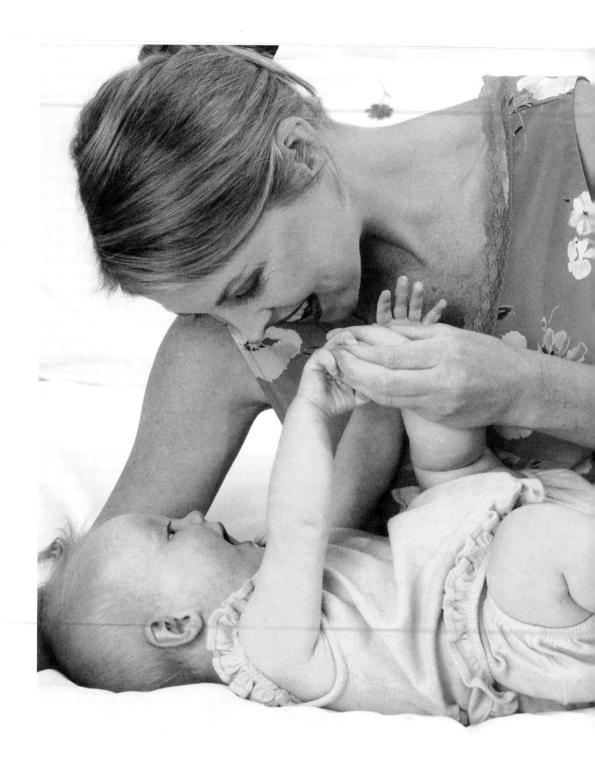

Conclusion

Just as every mother and baby is different, so is every mother and baby's feeding experience. Some will find breastfeeding easy and want it to go on for ever; others will find it harder and encounter problems. Some mothers will begin by breastfeeding and change to formula feeding early on; others will formula feed their baby from the start. Some mothers will find their experience changes completely from one baby to the next.

But whatever you experience, it is worth remembering that the amount of time your baby is entirely dependent upon you for her food is not long. Any problems or concerns you may have, can usually be overcome with patience and perseverance so that this short time of feeding your baby can be a joy and a time of the day that the two of you can look forward to with pleasure.

USEFUL ORGANISATIONS

Association of Breastfeeding Mothers
ABM
PO Box 207
BRIDGWATER
Somerset
TA6 7YT
Counselling Hotline: 08444 122 949
Website: www.abm.me.uk
Telephone advice service for breastfeeding mothers.

La Leche League (Great Britain)
PO Box 29
West Bridgford
Nottingham
NG2 7NP
Phone: 0845 456 1855 (Mondays and Thursdays, answerphone at other times)
Website: www.laleche.org.uk
Personal counselling and local groups to give help and information to women who want to breastfeed.

National Childbirth Trust (NCT)
The National Childbirth Trust
Alexandra House
Oldham Terrace
Acton
London
W3 6NH
General enquiry line: 0870 770 3236
Breastfeeding line: 0870 444 8708
(9am to 6pm, seven days a week) To talk to a qualified breastfeeding counsellor about breastfeeding.
Website: www.nct.org.uk
Antenatal and postnatal classes giving information and help to mothers, including help with breastfeeding.

Tamba
2 The Willows
Gardner Road
Guildford
GU1 4PG
Phone: 0870 770 3305
Website: www.tamba.org.uk
A nationwide UK charity providing information and mutual support networks for families of twins, triplets and more.

Twinsclub
PO Box 9494
Redditch
B98 8PQ
Website: www.twinsclub.co.uk
The UK-based multiples website for parents, and parents-to-be, of twins, triplets, quads and more.

INDEX

INDEX

1 3 5 7 9 10 8 6 4 2

Published in 2008 by Vermilion, an imprint of Ebury Publishing

A Random House Group Company

Copyright © Naia Edwards 2008

All photographs © Photolibrary Group

Naia Edwards has asserted her right to be identified as the author of this Work in accordance with the Copyright, Designs and Patents Act 1988

The Random House Group Limited Reg. No. 954009

Addresses for companies within the Random House Group can be found at www.randomhouse.co.uk

A CIP catalogue record for this book is available from the British Library

The Random House Group Limited makes every effort to ensure that the papers used in our books are made from trees that have been legally sourced from well-managed and credibly certified forests. Our paper procurement policy can be found on www.rbooks.co.uk/environment

To buy books by your favourite authors and register for offers visit www.rbooks.co.uk

Printed and bound in Singapore by Tien Wah Press

ISBN 9780091923433

Please note that conversions to imperial weights and measures are suitable equivalents and not exact.

The information given in this book should not be treated as a substitute for qualified medical advice; always consult a medical practitioner. Neither the author nor the publisher can be held responsible for any loss or claim arising out of the use, or misuse, of the suggestions made or the failure to take medical advice.